MEDICAL BILLING AND CODING 2024 – 2025

Maximize Your Career Potential with the Latest Trends, Certification Tips, and Industry Insights

George Sarah

Copyright@2024 George Sarah

All Rights Reserved

No part of this written publication may be reproduced, distributed, or shared in any form or by any means, including photocopying, recording, or other electronic or mechanical methods, without the publisher's prior written permission.

Contents

INTRODUCTION 1

CHAPTER ONE: WHAT IS MEDICAL BILLING AND CODING 1

TYPES OF CODING 3

    ICD 3

    CPT 3

    HCPCS 4

WHY SHOULD WE CODE? 5

WHY WE BILL 5

IS MEDICAL BILLING DIFFERENT FROM MEDICAL CODING 6

IS MEDICAL BILLING AND CODING A DIFFICULT FIELD OF HEALTHCARE TO GET INTO? 7

IMPORTANCE OF MEDICAL BILLING AND CODING 8

MAKING YOUR BILLING AND CODING CAREER ENJOYABLE 9

CHAPTER TWO: MEDICAL ACCOUNTING AND JOB CODING PROSPECT ... 9

VALUE OF THE MEDICAL ACCOUNTING ROLE 10

MEDICAL ACCOUNTING AND GENERAL ACCOUNTING. HOW IS IT DIFFERENT? 10

HIPAA 11

Overview of HIPAA 11

    1. HIPAA Privacy Rule 11

    2. HIPAA Security Rule 12

    3. HIPAA Enforcement Rule 12

    4. HIPAA Breach Notification Rule 12

    5. HIPAA Omnibus Rule 13

Key Concepts and Definitions 13

    Covered Entities and Business Associates 13

    Protected Health Information (PHI) 13

    De-identified Information 14

    Compliance and Best Practices 14

    Enforcement and Penalties 14

JOB CODING PROSPECT 15

GETTING A JOB AS A MEDICAL CODER 15

CHAPTER THREE: WHAT ARE THE MEDICAL BILLING AND CODING CLASSES REQUIRED? 16

MEDICAL BILLING AND CODING: CORE CURRICULUM 17

    Terminology in Medicine 17

    Medical Procedures in the Office 17

    Body Systems I and II 17

    Pharmacology 17

    Health Insurance and Medical Billing 17

    HIPAA, Medical Contracts, and Ethics 17

    Coding for Hospital Applications/Medical Billing in Hospitals 18

    Coding for Medical Office Applications/Physician Medical Billing 18

    ICD-9 and ICD-10 Coding Basics 18

    Scenarios for Advanced Medical Coding 18

CERTIFICATION AND CERTIFYING BODIES 18

CHAPTER FOUR: WHAT DOES A SPECIALIST IN MEDICAL BILLING AND CODING DO? 19

CAN ONE PERSON TAKE UP BOTH JOBS 20
CHAPTER FIVE: HOW TO BECOME A MEDICAL BILLER AND CODER 20
BECOMING A MEDICAL CODER 21
WORK EXPERIENCE 22
ADVANCED MEDICAL CODING CERTIFICATIONS 22
    Certified Professional Coder (CPC) 22
    Certified Outpatient Coder (COC) 22
    Certified Inpatient Coder (CIC) 23
    Certified Risk Adjustment Coder (CRC) 23
CAREER ADVANCEMENT 24
BECOMING A MEDICAL BILLER 27
CHAPTER SIX: WHAT ARE THE QUALIFICATIONS FOR A SPECIALIST IN MEDICAL BILLING AND CODING? 28
CERTIFICATION ORGANIZATION 29
    American Academy of Professional Coders 29
    American Health Information Management Association (AHIMA) 29
    The Healthcare Billing and Management Association 30
    Medical Billers' Association (MAB) 31
    The Professional Association of Healthcare Coding Specialists 31
    Medical Specialty Coding and Compliance Board (BMSC) 31
MEDICAL BILLING AND CODING CERTIFICATION 32
    CERTIFICATION REQUIREMENTS 32
    HOW IMPORTANT ARE CERTIFICATIONS 33
MEDICAL BILLING AND CODING SKILLS 34

CHAPTER SEVEN: HOW TO SELECT AND PREPARE FOR CERTIFICATION MEDICAL CODE 36

SELECTING THE RIGHT CERTIFICATION 37

CHAPTER EIGHT: HOW LONG WILL IT TAKE TO BE A MEDICAL CODER? 38

IS MEDICAL BILLING AND CODING THE RIGHT CAREER FOR YOU? 38

CHAPTER NINE: REASONS TO BEGIN A CAREER IN MEDICAL BILLING AND CODING 39

CONCLUSION 42

INTRODUCTION

In most medical facilities across the country, doctors and nurses seem to be in charge. It is reasonable to think this because they are the ones who help people. At the same time, a lot of people work in hospitals, medical centers, and other health centers to make it possible for people to go to the doctor. This kind of work includes things like medical coding and billing.

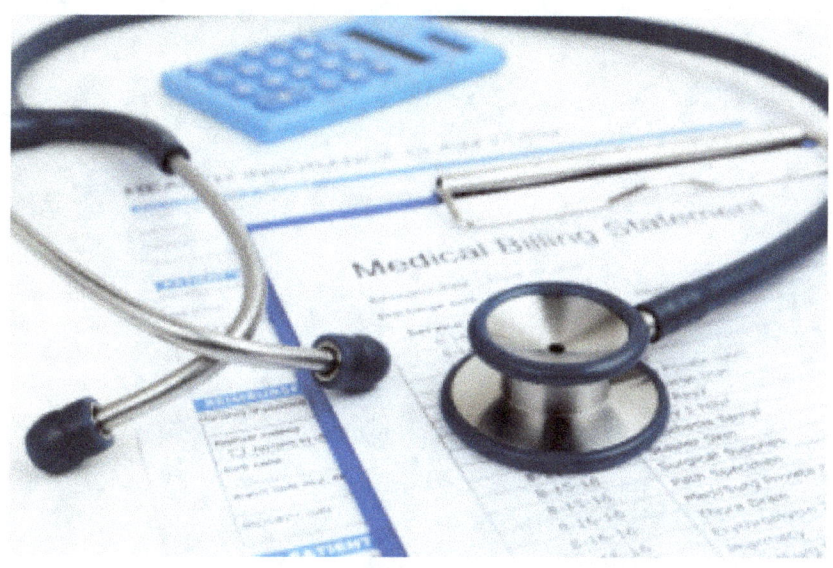

Medical billing is an important part of how well any hospital or medical facility runs. Writing up and sending insurance companies billing cases is part of medical billing. This makes sure that the hospital or medical office gets paid the right amount for the services they provide to customers.

Commercial insurance companies and some government-run healthcare programs help medical offices stay open. How long the medical office can stay open depends on how much money it brings in. Because they don't get paid enough, these organizations can't give people the best care possible.

Medical coding services came about because of the need to keep everything in order in a clear and organized way. When medical evaluations, medical services, and technology are turned into a set of alphanumeric medical numbers, this process is called medical coding. This explanation makes sure that records are kept consistently and helps administrators figure out how well and how common the treatment is.

CHAPTER ONE: WHAT IS MEDICAL BILLING AND CODING

Medical coding and billing are two parts of the current healthcare system that are linked in a way that can't be separated. Both of these things are important parts of the payment cycle that make sure healthcare workers get paid for their work. At this point, let's keep things easy and separate the two. Think of them as separate parts of a bigger process. First, let's talk about medical coding.

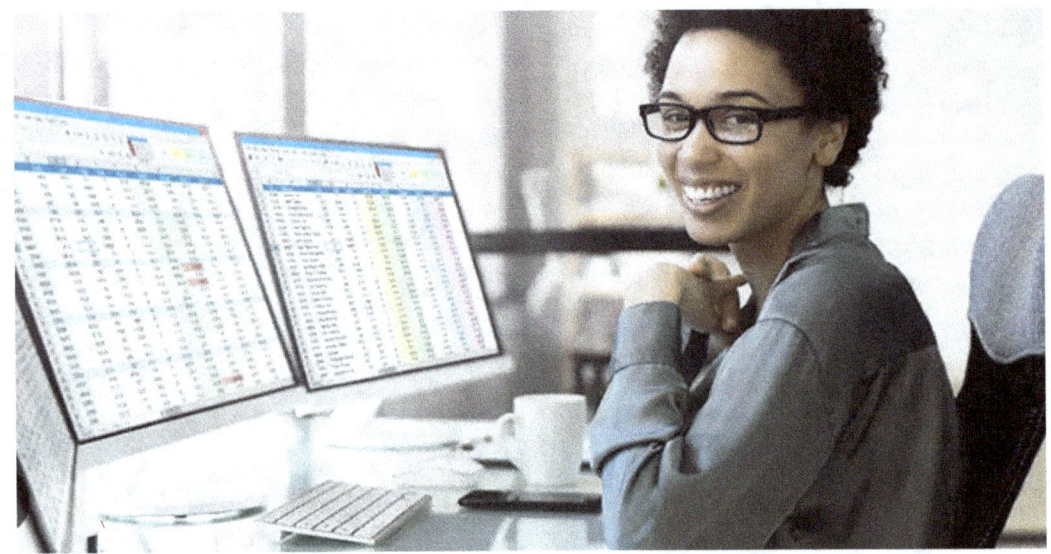

Medical Coding

Medical coding is similar to translation at its most basic level. The coder's job is to turn anything written in one way, like a doctor's report or an order for a certain drug, into a code that is made up of numbers or letters as accurately as possible. It has a number for every kind of accident, illness, and medical care.

There are tens of thousands of numbers for medical practices, minor treatments, and illnesses. To begin, let us look at a simple example of medical coding.

A person with whooping cough, a fever, and a lot of sputum or mucus comes to the doctor's office. After the nurse asks about the patient's symptoms and does some basic tests, the doctor checks them out and says they have bronchitis. After that, the doctor gives the patient medicine.

Every part of this meeting is written down by the doctor or someone from the healthcare provider's office. It is the job of the medical coder to turn all the important details from a patient's visit into numbers and alphabetical codes that can be used for billing. A medical coder needs to know a lot of different sets and groups of numbers.

When the doctor writes up a patient's visit report, the coder reads it and turns each piece of information into a code. A certain code is used for each type of visit, each patient's complaints, each test the doctor does, and each conclusion the doctor makes.

There are rules for every set of standards and norms. Some numbers, like those that show a pre-existing condition, need to be put in a certain order. Accurately coding and following the rules for each code will affect the legality of a claim.

Once a medical coder enters the correct numbers into a piece of software, the coding process is finished. Once the report has been coded, it is sent to the medical biller.

Medical Billing

On a single level, medical billing is exactly what it sounds like medical billers get the paperwork from the medical coder and make a claim for the insurance company. Like most things that have to do with health care, the process isn't as easy as it looks.

To get a better idea of what medical billing is, let's look at the last case again. The same patient is sneezing, has a fever, and is making a lot of mucus. This person calls the doctor to set up an appointment. This is the beginning of the medical billing process.

The medical biller gathers the numbers that represent the type of visit, the patient's symptoms, the doctor's diagnosis, and the doctor's medications and uses software to create a claim out of them. After that, the biller sends the claim to the insurance company. The insurance company looks it over and sends it back to the biller. The biller looks over the returned claim and decides how much of the bill the patient pays after the insurance is taken out.

If a person with bronchitis has insurance that covers this type of visit and care for this illness, our fee will be pretty low. The person might have to pay a copay or have made other plans with their insurance company. The biller looks at all the information and then makes a correct bill that is sent to the patient.

The medical biller might have to call a debt-collecting agency if a customer is late or refuses to pay the bill. This is to make sure that the healthcare provider gets paid.

So, the medical biller acts as a link between the customer, the healthcare provider, and the insurance company. You can think of the biller as an interpreter, just like the coder. The coder turns medical processes into codes, and the biller turns codes into financial records. While the biller does many things, for now, all you need to know is that their main job is to make sure the healthcare provider gets paid for their services.

TYPES OF CODING

As a medical coder, you'll use three different sets of codes regularly.

ICD

They are called ICD numbers, which stand for "**International Classification of Diseases.**" There is a normal way to talk about the reasons for illness, harm, and death with these diagnosis numbers.

In the late 1940s, the World Health Organization (WHO) made this set of codes. It has been changed many times in the more than 60 years since it began. The number after "ICD" tells you what version of the code is being used at the moment.

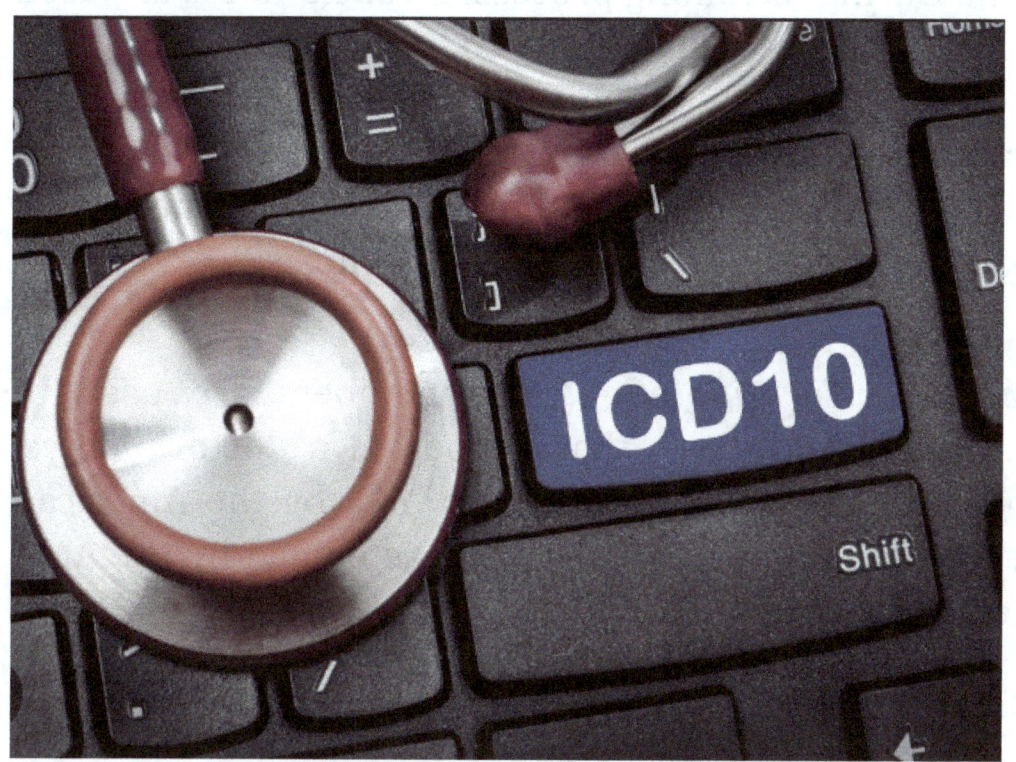

One code that is now used in the United States is ICD-10-CM. This means that this is the tenth version of the ICD code. The "-CM" at the end stands for "clinical modification." The full name for this number is the International Classification of Diseases, Tenth Revision, Clinical Modification. A group of changes called clinical modification (CMS) have been made by the National Center for Health Statistics (NCHS), which is part of the Center for Medicare and Medicaid Studies.

There are a lot more diagnostic codes now that the Clinical Modification has been made. This wider reach gives hackers a lot more options and accuracy, which are both very important in their job. The fact that there are 14,000 numbers in the ICD-10 system shows how important clinical change is. Its clinical form, ICD-10-CM, has almost 68,000 numbers.

People use ICD numbers to talk about both the diagnosis and the state of a patient. During the billing process, these numbers are used to show that a medical necessity exists. Coders have to make sure that the procedure they're billing for fits with the patient's description. Back to our strep throat example, a claim would almost certainly be turned down if a coder said that an x-ray was necessary for medical reasons because of a strep throat diagnosis.

CPT

Current Procedural Terminology (CPT) numbers are used to record most medical procedures that happen in a doctor's office. This set of codes is put out and kept up to date by the American Medical Association (AMA). These numbers are owned by the AMA and are updated every year.

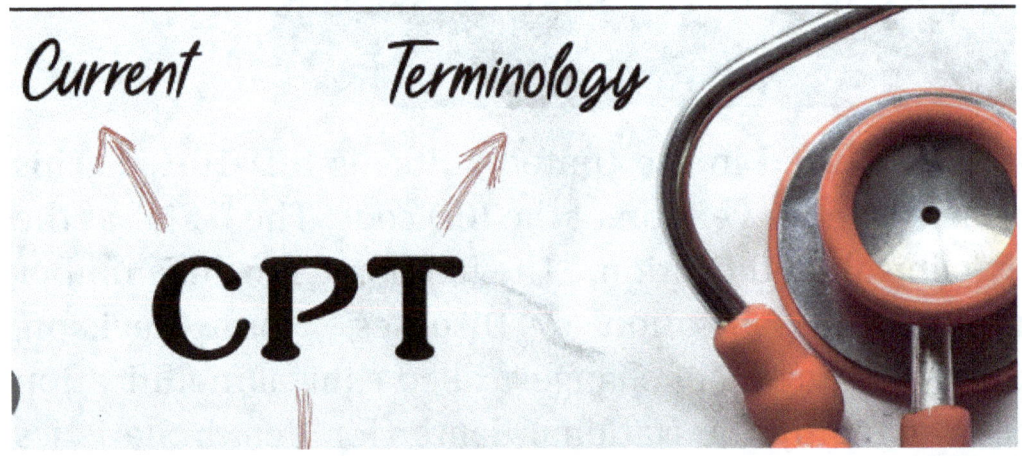

The five-digit numbers that makeup CPT codes are split into three groups. People most often use the first group, which is made up of six groups. In this range, there are six main medical specialties: evaluation and management, anesthesia, surgery, radiology, pathology, the lab, and medicine.

In the second group are CPT numbers for performance reviews and, in some cases, results from lab or x-ray tests. They are generally put at the end of a Category I CPT code with a space. The codes are made up of five numbers and letters.

You don't have to use Category II numbers; you can use Category I codes instead. The **American Medical Association (AMA)** says that these codes will help other doctors and medical professionals. The AMA also says that Category II codes will make doctors' offices less busy by giving them more and more accurate information about how well health professionals and health facilities are doing.

A third group of CPT numbers stands for "emerging medical technology." As a coder, you'll spend most of your time on the first two groups, but the first one will probably come up more often.

There are also addendums to CPT codes that make them more precise and right. The American Medical Association (AMA) made a set of CPT modifications because the normal Category I CPT code doesn't give enough information for some medical treatments.

There are two-digit numbers or alphabetic codes that come after the CPT code for Category I. These codes give more information about the process code, which makes it more valuable. For instance, there is a CPT tag that tells you which side of the body an operation is done on, and there is also a code for an ended surgery.

HCPCS

The **Healthcare Common Procedure Coding System (HCPCS)** is a set of codes that are built on the CPT numbers. It is usually said as "hick picks." The American Medical Association manages HCPCS codes, which were made by the CMS (the same organization that made CPT). Most of them have to do with tasks, methods, and tools that aren't covered by CPT codes. Some examples are large medical centers, replacements, rescue rides, and certain meds and treatments.

HCPCS is the official code system for a lot of different services, not just outpatient hospital care, treatment drugs, Medicaid, and Medicare. Because they are used by both Medicaid and Medicare, HCPCS codes are some of the most important ones that a medical writer can use.

The HCPCS coding set is made up of two levels. The first level is the same as the CPT numbers we already talked about.

Level II is made up of a list of numerical codes that are grouped into 17 groups. Each group focuses on a different area of skill, like medical and testing services or therapeutic services.

Both CPT and HCPCS numbers should have a diagnosis code that goes with them to explain the medical process. The coders' job is to make sure that the outpatient procedure discussed by the doctor in the statement matches the given illness, which is usually described with an ICD code.

You should have a better idea of what each of these codes does now.

WHY SHOULD WE CODE?

First, a simple question about medical coding: Why do medical notes need to be coded? After writing down the symptoms, diagnosis, and treatments, wouldn't it be enough to just send them to health insurance and wait to see what services they cover?

The Centers for Disease Control and Prevention (CDC) said that 1.4 billion patients had been seen in 2018. Trips to hospital care centers, doctor's offices, and emergency rooms are included in this number. Even if we only assume that each visit sends five bits of coded information, which is a very low number, that's six billion unique pieces of data every year. Medical coding makes it possible to send big amounts of data easily in a world where there is a lot of it.

Coding also makes it easier for medical institutions to keep notes that are the same. They both use the same code for a streptococcal sore throat. Standardized data makes it easier to evaluate and ask questions, which the government and medical institutions can use to keep an eye on health trends. If the CDC wants to find out how often viral pneumonia happens, for example, they could use the ICD-10-CM number to look at all the new cases of pneumonia.

Last but not least, medical coding companies let facility managers check how often and how well treatment is working. Twelfth-level hospitals and other large medical facilities need to know this. Medical institutions may figure out how well they're doing by looking at data, in the same way that the government keeps track of how often a disease happens.

WHY WE BILL

Going to the doctor may seem like a one-on-one interaction, but it's part of a large, complex system for sharing information and making payments. The covered person can only work with one person or medical expert, but the check-up is part of a three-party scheme.

The patient is the first person involved. This is the second party: the medical expert. Any place that offers health services, like hospitals, doctors' offices, physiotherapy studios, emergency rooms, outpatient care centers, and more, is called a supplier. The third and last party is the insurance company, also called the payer.

The medical biller's job is to talk about and work out payments between these three groups. The biller ensures that the medical provider receives payment for their services by billing both customers and payers. We charge because people who work in health care need to be paid for the services they provide.

To do this, the biller puts together a bill for the insurance company by putting together all the paperwork (in the form of a "superbill") about the patient and the surgery that was done on them. A claim is a bill that lists the patient's name, address, health information, and insurance benefits. It also includes a report of the treatments that were given and why they were done.

IS MEDICAL BILLING DIFFERENT FROM MEDICAL CODING

There are a lot of people who think that medical billing and medical coding are the same thing, but they are not. If you don't know any better, these two jobs may look the same, but they are very different. The experts in both fields use similar skills to get similar results, but their methods and ways of reaching their goals are very different.

These two sets of skills are similar because they both involve translating medical paperwork into controlled codes so that important health information can be sent from one person to another. Medical billers are concerned with making sure that patients get paid correctly and on time-based on the codes that are used. A medical coder's job is to give the most complete picture of a clinical interaction possible, leaving the financial details to the billers.

When medical bills are sent in, medical billers usually work with patients and insurance companies. Most of the time, billers care more about the customer than medical coders do. Medical coders usually work with healthcare workers to make sure that the services and goods given to patients are properly categorized. Please see the table below for some of the main differences between medical billing and coding:

MEDICAL BILLING	MEDICAL CODING
It mostly involves entering information into billing software.	To identify the services given to a patient, you need to talk to doctors, nurses, and other health care workers.
Putting together insurance claims and sending them to insurance companies.	Standardized numbers from CPT, HCPCS, and ICD-10 CM are used on patient data to accurately show the services that were provided.
Follow up with patients, medical workers, and insurance companies to make sure bills are paid.	Electronic medical record (EMR) and electronic health record (EHR) software are used to enter data in hospitals and doctors' offices.
Keep track of bills and account payments	Going over operation reports to make sure diagnosis codes were used correctly during surgery
Looking at claims that have been turned down or refused	When a claim is turned down, they do checks of the medical

	charts.
Making sure that insurance companies pay doctors and people back	It is very important to stay up to date on the latest changes to government rules and coding standards.
Make sure that the personal health information numbers that medical writers use to group services and things are right.	Checking that the coding correctly describes a patient's medical care by looking over their data and backgrounds.

IS MEDICAL BILLING AND CODING A DIFFICULT FIELD OF HEALTHCARE TO GET INTO?

NO, it's not! It might look like medical billing and coding is hard and complicated, but it might not be as hard as you think. As long as you get the right training, education, and practice, medical billing and coding can be a fun and rewarding job.

There are challenges in medical billing and coding, just like in any other job. These challenges are especially hard for people who are new to the field. Many people who work in medical billing and coding say that the three biggest problems they face are:

The Language: Medical Billing and Coding Specialists use one of three main coding systems to find medical signs and treatments and write them down. When you look at these three coding schemes, it's easy to think that you are learning a new language. But coders can get help in the form of reference books and useful apps, which makes learning about coding much easier.

But coders can get help in the form of reference books and useful apps, which makes learning about coding much easier.

Details: Sorting medical signs or treatments into groups often involves a lot of steps, and a lot of different things need to be looked at. It might be hard to remember everything that needs to be done for each task. Taking care of all the little details is a lot easier once you have the right knowledge and tools.

The equipment: Medical Billing and Coding Specialists use high-tech coding tools to do their jobs. Because this technology is usually complicated, it might be hard to learn, understand, and use. If the Specialist has the right training and experience, these tools are an important part of their job.

These may look like big problems, but most Medical Billing and Coding Specialists can solve them without any trouble and go on to have long, satisfying jobs.

IMPORTANCE OF MEDICAL BILLING AND CODING

Two of the best things about any healthcare center are medical billing and coding. The health of the public, getting paid on time, and running a business smoothly all rest on correctness in these areas. People who work in medical billing and coding need to be highly skilled and able to quickly read, analyze, record, and handle difficult medical data while protecting client privacy and paying close attention to detail.

It's become more important for people who can work in billing and coding as the medical field has grown.

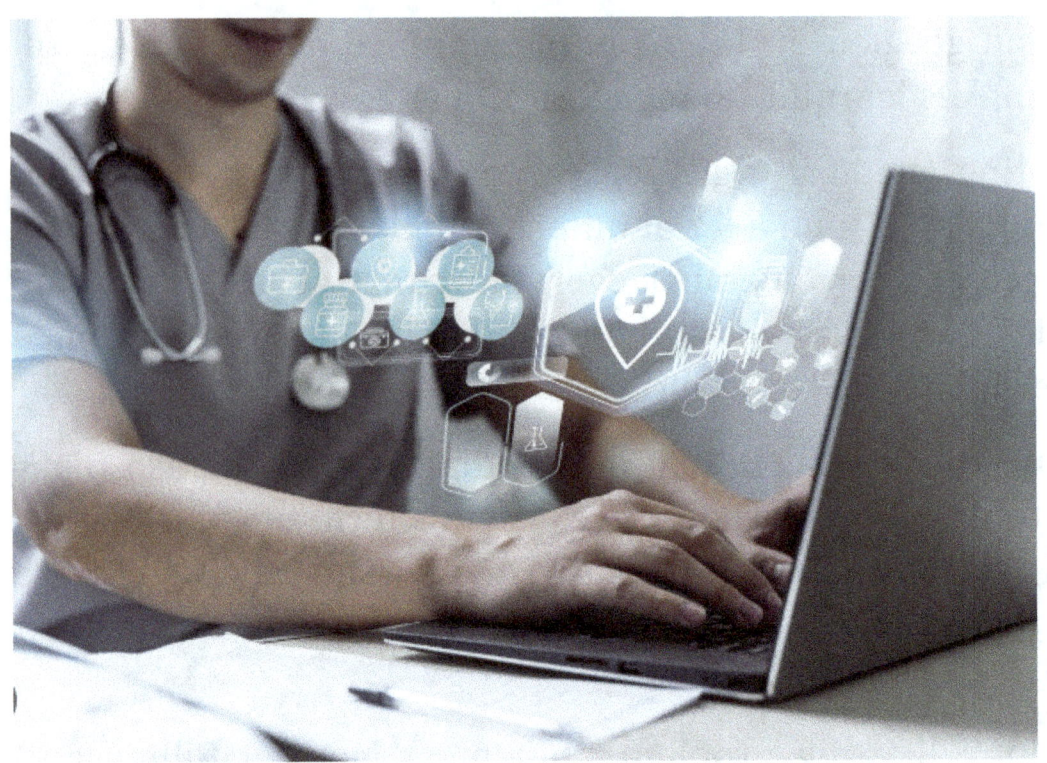

Medical practices and businesses need people who are experts in medical billing and coding. Services that do medical billing and coding are very important for connecting customers with doctors or medical groups. It is the job of a medical billing and coding expert to connect these three groups:

The Patient, The Medical Institution, And The Insurance Company

The person who does the billing and coding makes sure that bills, data, and other tasks are done on time. One of their major jobs is to handle health insurance and refund cases. They are also responsible for coding medical records, diagnostic tests, and other data related to patient claims.

When doctors and offices hire someone to do medical billing and coding, they often get more than one benefit. If they hire a medical billing and coding expert, it might save them a lot of trouble with management.

This area of work is growing, which is good news for many reasons. People who work in this field can do their jobs from home and get paid well, which is a big plus. Another benefit is that online jobs can be very profitable in today's world where everything is pretty much on the Internet. It's the same in the world of medical coding and billing!

Medical billing and coding are important because they affect medical care in a roundabout way, especially when it comes to getting paid by insurance. In today's fee-for-service medical market, doctors are expected to explain underlying diseases, unsolved diagnoses, and basic standards more and more. Medical coding makes sure that insurance companies have all the medical numbers they need to pay the right amount of money. Coding is required for a variety of purposes, including demographic studies, disease incidence research, treatment outcomes, and responsible and open payment systems.

MAKING YOUR BILLING AND CODING CAREER ENJOYABLE

- **Dedicate yourself to learning**: Students who only know the basics of the material may find it hard to deal with the problems it brings up. Learn as much as you can about billing and coding, even if you already have a job. You might learn something new that will make or break your job.
- **Keep your information up to date**. Because healthcare changes so quickly and often, it's important to know the latest rules and laws for coding and billing. To learn more about the field, read trade magazines, regularly ask your bosses for information, and make connections with other people in the same field.

- **Difficulties in research and review**: You'll be better able to handle your problems if you know more about them. When you have a problem, you should think about how to fix it. It's likely that the next time you have a problem like this, it will be a lot easier.

CHAPTER TWO: MEDICAL ACCOUNTING AND JOB CODING PROSPECT

Like many other jobs in the health field, medical billing and coding are becoming more popular. The BLS predicts that by 2026, there will be 22% more jobs for healthcare workers, which includes people who do medical billing and coding. This rate is a lot higher than the national average, and it will mean that 129,000 more jobs will be open in the next few years.

According to the current job market, medical billing and coding might be a good choice if predicted job openings are important to your work goals. As the population ages, more people will need medical services. There will be more medical record changes and insurance claims to handle because of the rise in these services.

If you work in medical billing and coding, more medical claims could mean more people needing your skills and experience. Everyone who needs to fill out a medical claim would have to organize and code all of the information.

Also, medical companies will need trained workers who know how to use this technology a lot because they are quickly becoming dependent on computer tools to run their businesses. After you finish your training and get your license, the faster job growth in this field should make you feel good about your long-term job chances.

VALUE OF THE MEDICAL ACCOUNTING ROLE

Particularly if you work in the healthcare business, you've probably heard of medical billing and accounting and have a general idea of what they mean. On the other hand, a lot of people don't understand what medical billing and accounting are and often mix them up with medical transcription or medical coding. But all three are different from each other.

They are indeed linked. To be clear, though, medical transcription only involves typing up doctor's notes, while medical coding is only about writing down codes. As part of a managed services system, the medical accounting and billing system handles front-desk tasks, insurance claims, and money matters, and has a strong focus on billing and medical accounting. More chores go into medical accounting and billing than into medical transcription and coding.

For example, working at the front desk comes with more duties and roles than one might first think. For example, you may have to be the executive assistant for the practice and do secretarial tasks like registering patients, making sure appointments are kept, recording hospital records, writing down how diagnoses and treatments are carried out, and using software to organize health records.

The first time a patient comes to the office, the person in charge of accounting and billing will take care of everything, from making sure the patient arrives on time to setting up meetings. Based on the services provided and the review, the doctor will create and change the patient's medical record after seeing them. They put these facts in order using a method that has been used before in practice.

MEDICAL ACCOUNTING AND GENERAL ACCOUNTING. HOW IS IT DIFFERENT?

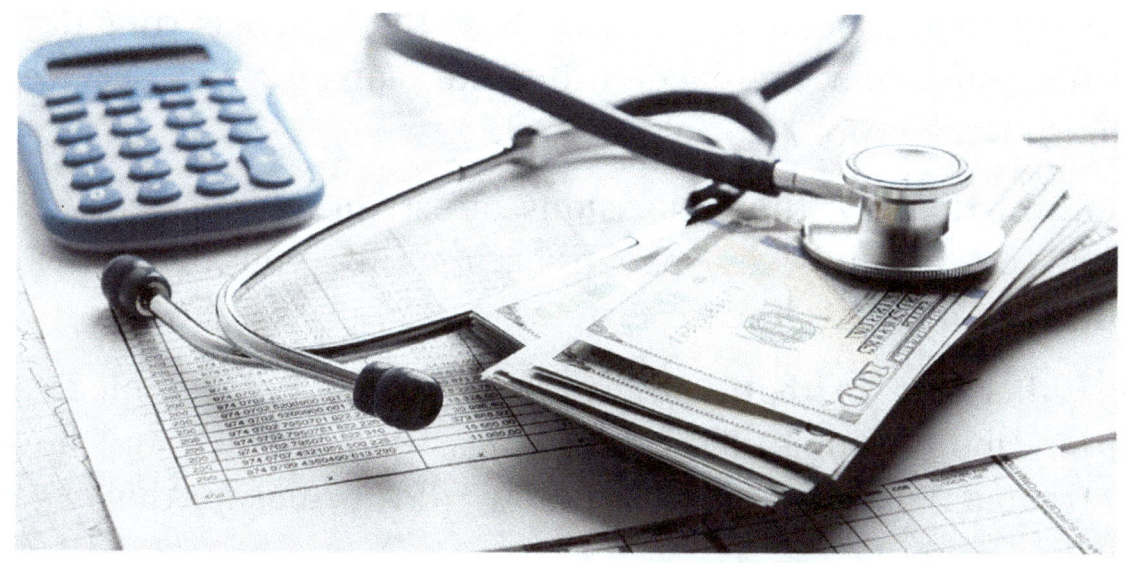

In general accounting, which is what the name suggests, you record and make financial accounts of all kinds of transactions, like bank fees debit, and credits. You also keep track of your income for the current fiscal or calendar year. This process is linked to the general work of a business account, organization, or group, as well as to non-profits and government agencies.

Many things go into general accounting, but the most important thing is keeping general accounting records on ledgers and supervising as needed. For example, you might be in charge of grants accounting or ledger accounts for post-retirement and pension funds.

Accounting for healthcare facilities is all about keeping track of what's going on in the hospital or clinic. This means they need to know how much money is coming in and going out. Healthcare companies must also follow the rules when it comes to taxes and audits. These rules are often hard to understand. Because of this, they need someone with a lot of knowledge in this field who can work with their rules.

Healthcare accountants are in charge of both of these tasks. In turn, this helps the leaders of the service or group make better decisions. These decisions may sometimes affect how the business runs day-to-day. Sometimes they are needed to make plans for new services and actions in the future.

At the end of the day, these decisions affect the people who use these services. In this way, as an accountant, you become an important part of the healthcare system.

One big difference is that you can always see private medical information about people, like what illnesses they have and how they are treated. You would have to follow HIPAA rules for this.

HIPAA

The Health Insurance Portability and Accountability Act (HIPAA) is a significant piece of legislation in the United States, enacted in 1996. It addresses the protection and confidential handling of protected health information (PHI). HIPAA has two primary purposes: to provide continuous health insurance coverage for workers who lose or change their jobs and to reduce the administrative burdens and cost of healthcare by standardizing the electronic transmission of administrative and financial transactions. However, one of the most critical aspects of HIPAA is its rules concerning the privacy and security of health information.

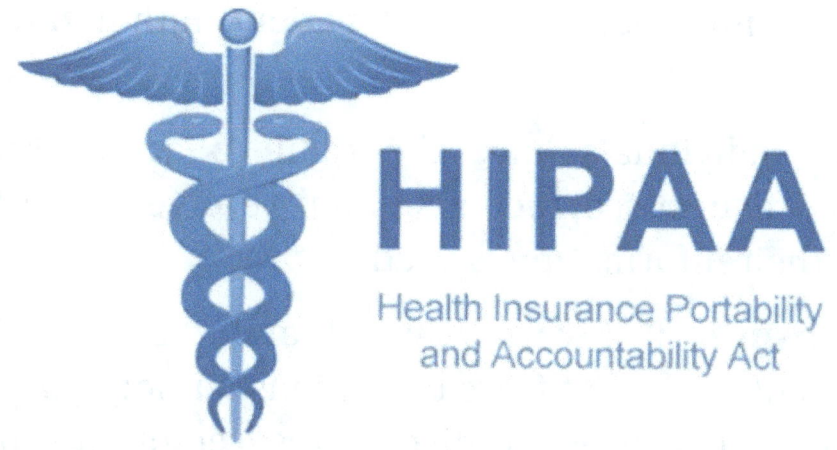

Overview of HIPAA

HIPAA consists of several key components:

1. **HIPAA Privacy Rule**
2. **HIPAA Security Rule**
3. **HIPAA Enforcement Rule**
4. **HIPAA Breach Notification Rule**
5. **HIPAA Omnibus Rule**

Each of these components plays a vital role in protecting PHI and ensuring that healthcare entities comply with the standards set by HIPAA.

1. HIPAA Privacy Rule

The HIPAA Privacy Rule establishes national standards to protect individuals' medical records and other personal health information. It applies to health plans, healthcare clearinghouses, and healthcare providers that conduct certain healthcare transactions electronically. The Privacy Rule requires appropriate safeguards to protect the privacy of PHI and sets limits and conditions on the uses and disclosures of such information without patient authorization. Key provisions include:

- **Patient Rights:** Individuals have the right to access their health records, request corrections, and receive a notice explaining how their information is used.

- **Use and Disclosure:** PHI can be used and disclosed for treatment, payment, and healthcare operations without patient consent, but any other uses or disclosures require explicit authorization.

- **Minimum Necessary Standard:** When using or disclosing PHI, covered entities must make reasonable efforts to ensure that only the minimum necessary information is shared.

2. HIPAA Security Rule

The HIPAA Security Rule specifies safeguards that covered entities and their business associates must implement to protect the confidentiality, integrity, and availability of electronic protected health information (ePHI). It focuses on three types of safeguards:

- **Administrative Safeguards:** Policies and procedures designed to manage the selection, development, implementation, and maintenance of security measures to protect ePHI.

- **Physical Safeguards:** Measures to protect electronic information systems and related buildings and equipment from natural and environmental hazards and unauthorized intrusion.

- **Technical Safeguards:** Technology and the policy and procedures for its use that protect ePHI and control access to it.

3. HIPAA Enforcement Rule

The HIPAA Enforcement Rule establishes procedures for investigating and resolving potential violations of HIPAA standards. It outlines the penalties for non-compliance, which can be significant. Penalties are tiered based on the level of negligence and can range from $100 to $50,000 per violation, with an annual maximum of $1.5 million. The Enforcement Rule also provides guidelines for compliance audits and investigations.

4. HIPAA Breach Notification Rule

The HIPAA Breach Notification Rule requires covered entities and business associates to provide notification following a breach of unsecured PHI. Notifications must be made to affected individuals, the Secretary of the U.S. Department of Health and Human Services (HHS), and, in certain circumstances, the media. Key elements include:

- **Breach Definition:** A breach is defined as the acquisition, access, use, or disclosure of PHI in a manner not permitted by the Privacy Rule, which compromises the security or privacy of the PHI.

- **Risk Assessment:** When a breach occurs, a risk assessment must be conducted to determine the potential harm and the likelihood that the PHI has been compromised.

- **Notification Requirements:** Notifications must be sent without unreasonable delay and no later than 60 days following the discovery of a breach.

5. HIPAA Omnibus Rule

The HIPAA Omnibus Rule, enacted in 2013, made several significant changes to the existing HIPAA regulations. It:

- **Strengthened Privacy and Security Protections:** The Omnibus Rule expanded the requirements for business associates and subcontractors to comply with HIPAA.

- **Increased Patient Rights:** Patients gained additional rights to request electronic copies of their health records and restrict disclosures to health plans.

- **Enhanced Enforcement:** The rule increased penalties for non-compliance and provided more stringent guidelines for breach notifications and risk assessments.

Key Concepts and Definitions

Covered Entities and Business Associates

- **Covered Entities:** Organizations subject to HIPAA regulations, including health plans, healthcare clearinghouses, and healthcare providers that transmit health information electronically.

- **Business Associates:** Individuals or entities that perform functions or activities on behalf of a covered entity involving the use or disclosure of PHI. Business associates are also subject to HIPAA regulations.

Protected Health Information (PHI)

PHI includes any information that relates to an individual's past, present, or future physical or mental health condition, the provision of healthcare, or the payment for healthcare. It includes common identifiers such as name, address, birth date, and Social Security number.

De-identified Information

De-identified information is health information that has been stripped of all identifying details, making it no longer subject to HIPAA regulations. De-identification can be achieved through two methods:

- **Safe Harbor Method:** Removing all 18 specified identifiers of the individual and their relatives, household members, and employers.
- **Expert Determination Method:** Having an expert apply statistical or scientific principles to determine that the risk of re-identification is very small.

Compliance and Best Practices

Compliance with HIPAA requires ongoing efforts to ensure that policies, procedures, and practices align with the regulatory requirements. Best practices for compliance include:

- **Conducting Risk Assessments:** Regularly assessing potential risks and vulnerabilities to ePHI and implementing appropriate safeguards.

- **Developing and Implementing Policies and Procedures:** Establishing clear policies and procedures for handling PHI, including privacy and security protocols.

- **Training and Awareness:** Providing regular training for employees and business associates on HIPAA requirements and the importance of protecting PHI.

- **Monitoring and Auditing:** Continuously monitoring access to PHI and conducting audits to ensure compliance with HIPAA standards.

- **Incident Response Planning:** Developing a plan for responding to security incidents and breaches, including notification procedures and mitigation strategies.

Enforcement and Penalties

Non-compliance with HIPAA can result in significant penalties, including:

- **Civil Penalties:** Fines ranging from $100 to $50,000 per violation, with an annual maximum of $1.5 million, depending on the level of negligence.

- **Criminal Penalties:** For more severe violations, individuals can face criminal penalties, including fines and imprisonment.

JOB CODING PROSPECT

Claim submission to insurance companies or the government is a part of medical coding. For the treatments to be paid for, the claims would need to include medical information of the patients.

For someone to get certified as a medical coding expert, they need to be able to do thorough work well, be comfortable with computers, want to work in health care and enjoy learning medical coding number codes. A medical writer also needs to have a strong sense of duty, work hard all the time, and be able to balance the need to keep medical data private.

After you finish your medical coding training, you can use what you've learned in different jobs. Billing supervisor, patient profile manager, health claims examiner, healthcare collector, payment expert, medical clinic helper, and medical claims handler are just a few of the many jobs that are currently being offered. They will only hire experienced writers or billers, which stresses how important it is to get certified.

GETTING A JOB AS A MEDICAL CODER

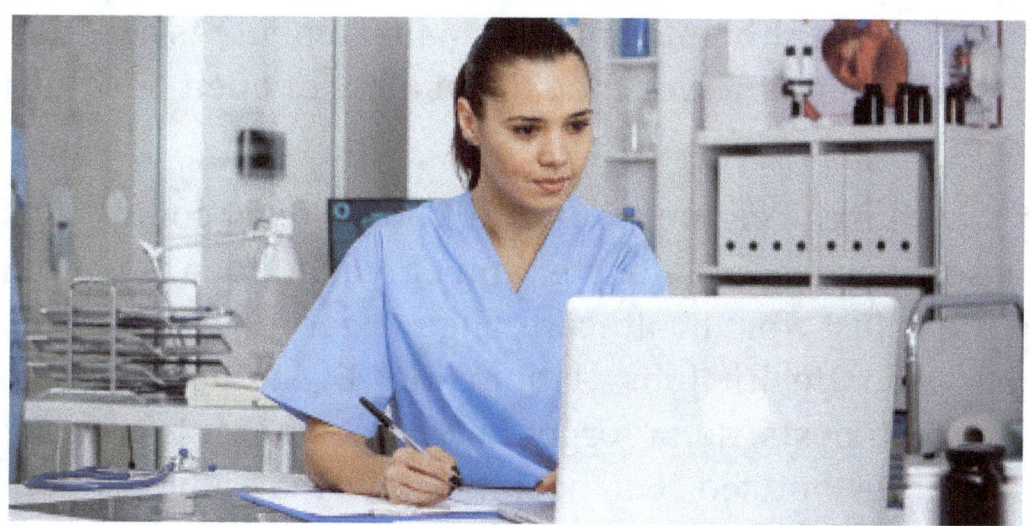

Begin your employment hunt as soon as possible. You shouldn't wait to look for work until you finish school. Use the services your school offers to help you find a job. Internships are a great way to meet new people and learn new things. You might want to do a job while you are still in school because many of them don't pay. You can also get experience and network by volunteering at a place where you want to work or asking to shadow an experienced medical writer. Before you look for a job, work on your resume and get feedback from someone else.

Consider taking a different path. If you can't find a job as a medical coder, you can always look for other jobs in the medical field to get your foot in the door. Think about working at the front desk or in the medical center. Because you have worked as a medical writer before, you are qualified for these jobs. You could ask the doctors, nurses, and other people you meet if they know of any open medical coding jobs.

Make contact with your professional association. The AHIMA and AAPC are great places to look for work. The AAPC has a job board and a program to help coders who are just getting qualified find work. Anyone who is a member of the AAPC can see all of these tools. The American Health Information Management Association (AHIMA) offers workshops, a workbook, and a list of open positions to help people prepare for their careers.

Make use of job search engines. You can find medical coding jobs on general job search sites like Monster and CareerBuilder as well as on sites that are just for healthcare, like Health Career Web, Biohealthmatics, and Health Jobs Nationwide. Even though these sites have a lot of job posts, don't forget how important it is to make relationships and get noticed. Let people know that you want to work as a medical coder. These big search engines shouldn't be the only places you look for job prospects.

Make sure you are prepared for the interview. If you want to get the job, you should research the company and be ready to talk about your skills. You have to also say why you want to work there and how your skills would help the company. You might be tested on how well you know medical terminology, electronic medical records, how to process claims, and how to use coding software. Talk about your job goals and any plans you have to get certified if you aren't already qualified. Make eye contact, give a firm handshake, and dress properly for your interview. Wear dress pants or skirts, blazers, coats, a dress shirt, or a top.

Make sure you're ready to take an exam. Some potential companies may want to see how well you can do on a skills test. There isn't a controlled test that everyone agrees on. You will be tested on how quickly, consistently, and carefully you pay attention to details, as well as how well you can choose the right numbers. To find out how long the test is and if you need to bring your coding books, you should ask.

CHAPTER THREE: WHAT ARE THE MEDICAL BILLING AND CODING CLASSES REQUIRED?

Medical coding offers classes leading to certificates, master's degrees, and associate's degrees. Most diploma programs in medical billing and coding are enough to get a job, and you can finish them in less than a year. Courses like these are often part of medical billing and coding programs:

1. Diagnostic Coding
2. Procedural Coding
3. Billing and Coding Application
4. Introduction to Computers
5. Introduction to Healthcare Communication
6. Medical Terminology
7. Medical Law and Ethics
8. Records Management
9. Healthcare Settings, Claim Cycle, and Claims Processing
10. Anatomy, Physiology, and Pathophysiology

Associate's degrees in medical coding take two years to finish and include a general studies component. Getting a better level of education, like an associate's degree, may open up more job possibilities. Some schools that teach medical coding may also help you get certain credentials after you finish, which could help you get a job.

Teaching assistantships, internships, and other types of hands-on work experience may be part of some schools, but they aren't always available or needed. There are a lot of online medical coding degree programs that can be done almost entirely online.

MEDICAL BILLING AND CODING: CORE CURRICULUM

The best classes in medical billing and coding cover both medical and administrative topics. The program includes things like anatomy, drugs, and medical terms. Then, they combine them with business needs, like keeping records. Specialists need to know about changes in the health care system, especially when it comes to privacy rules and billing for insurance. The following classes might be part of a medical billing and coding program:

Terminology in Medicine

People who aren't used to medical words, like long names for illnesses and short forms for medical numbers, might think it sounds like a different language. Students learn the basics and history of medical terms in these classes. They also learn how to study, describe, and create them.

Medical Procedures in the Office

As an administrative assistant, this class teaches students how to do things like answer the phone, sort digital and print mail, write professional letters, make plans for vacations and conferences, and schedule jobs in a medical setting.

Body Systems I and II

This set of studies gives students a real understanding of the human shape and the medical terms used to talk about how the body works. The vascular, muscular, and breathing systems are a few of them. Students also learn terms used in pharmacology and laboratories. The second course builds on the first by going into more depth about more difficult parts of the body and medical terms like genetics, cancer, and sense organs.

Pharmacology

Drugs have the power to kill or save lives. Do not let a medicine turn into a poison. Check the sticker to make sure the name, amount, and directions are right. Students learn about generic and brand-name medicines, as well as the side effects of drugs and how to mix medicines. They also look into how medicines affect different parts of the body.

Health Insurance and Medical Billing

This course for college freshmen talks about how to get different types of health insurance reimbursed and paid for. They learn about banking systems, charge plans, coding methods, and how to do a company check.

HIPAA, Medical Contracts, and Ethics

This course talks about different parts of health insurance plans and the services that are covered for patients, like preventative care and doctor visits. Ethics are also talked about, such as how to handle and share personal health information in line with the Health Insurance Portability and Accountability Act (HIPAA). It also has the electronic health record (EHR) benefits from the Health Information Technology for Economic and Clinical Health (HITECH) Act.

Coding for Hospital Applications/Medical Billing in Hospitals

Specialists in medical billing and coding usually work in places with a lot of patients and a lot of activity. The Centers for Disease Control and Prevention say that 130 million people went to emergency rooms in the US in 2011. This number does not include people who were moved to other medical areas. This is important for students to know: what is the difference between inpatient and outpatient care? How do I fill out regular hospital billing claim forms? Also, they need to be able to quickly make cases and follow up on them.

Coding for Medical Office Applications/Physician Medical Billing

Medical offices can work at the same speed as hospitals and use the same standard codes. In this class, students learn the right way to fill out medical claims forms, both by hand and on a computer. They use the CMS-1500 form, which is used for Medicare claims, to figure out why claims are being held up or turned down.

ICD-9 and ICD-10 Coding Basics

There is a shorthand-coded word for every disease, condition, sickness, diagnosis, and treatment. These numbers make it easier for medical billers to file claims and for doctors and nurses to keep track of the care they give to patients. Students learn how to code in ICD-9 and ICD-10 in this session. Expert coding is also taught for things like heart, pathology, and lab processes.

Medical Coding: Intermediate Students will learn how to use the CPT, ICD-9, and ICD-10 classification systems to code illnesses and processes in this lesson, which builds on the general coding skills course they took before.

Scenarios for Advanced Medical Coding

In the third level of studies, students use CPT, ICD-9, ICD-10, and HCPCS to give numbers in more complex medical coding cases. In this class, which builds on the basics and advanced studies, students will learn how to read and understand messy medical data. In addition, it helps them get ready for the CPC-A test.

CERTIFICATION AND CERTIFYING BODIES

Two groups that offer medical coding licensing are the American Academy of Professional Coders (AAPC) and the American Health Information Management Association (AHIMA). AHIA's two main certifications are the Certified Coding Associate (CCA) and the Certified Coding Specialist (CCS).

For the CCA, you need to finish a medical coding school or have been working as a coder for six months. For the CCS, you need two years of experience or the CCA certificate plus one more year of experience. People who want to get both diplomas must pass a licensing test.

The most well-known certification from the AAPC is the Certified Professional Coder (CPC) designation. An associate's degree is recommended but not required. For full designation, you need to have worked for two years. If you pass the test with less than two years of experience, you will be given the CPC-A (apprentice) certification until you meet the experience requirement.

There are also certificates for hospital, outpatient, and risk adjustment, as well as more than 20 certificates for specialists in areas such as general surgery, heart, and pediatrics. These specific credentials are meant to go along with the main titles that are already out there.

Some companies may want or even need certification as a way to show that you have the skills they're looking for. For most certifications, you need to keep learning to keep your certification. The requirements for continued education vary by certification.

Certifications facilitated by professional organizations include:

1. Certified Coding Specialist (CCS)
2. Certified Outpatient Coding (COC)
3. Certified Professional Biller (CPB)
4. Certified Billing and Coding Specialist (CBCS) from the National Health career Association
5. Certified Professional Coder (CPC)
6. Certified Coding Associate (CCA) from the American Health Information Management Association (AHIMA)
7. Certified Medical Coder (CMC) from the Practice Management Institute (PMI)

CHAPTER FOUR: WHAT DOES A SPECIALIST IN MEDICAL BILLING AND CODING DO?

An expert is someone who works between the insurance company and the doctor's office. People who work in the billing area of a healthcare group are called coding specialists, who are also sometimes called medical coders. These codes are very important for insurance billing, and one of their main jobs is to give each type of treatment a unique number that can be used for billing, studying, and keeping records. In the medical field, a coder might work for a clinic, a hospital, or even a study center for clinical trials.

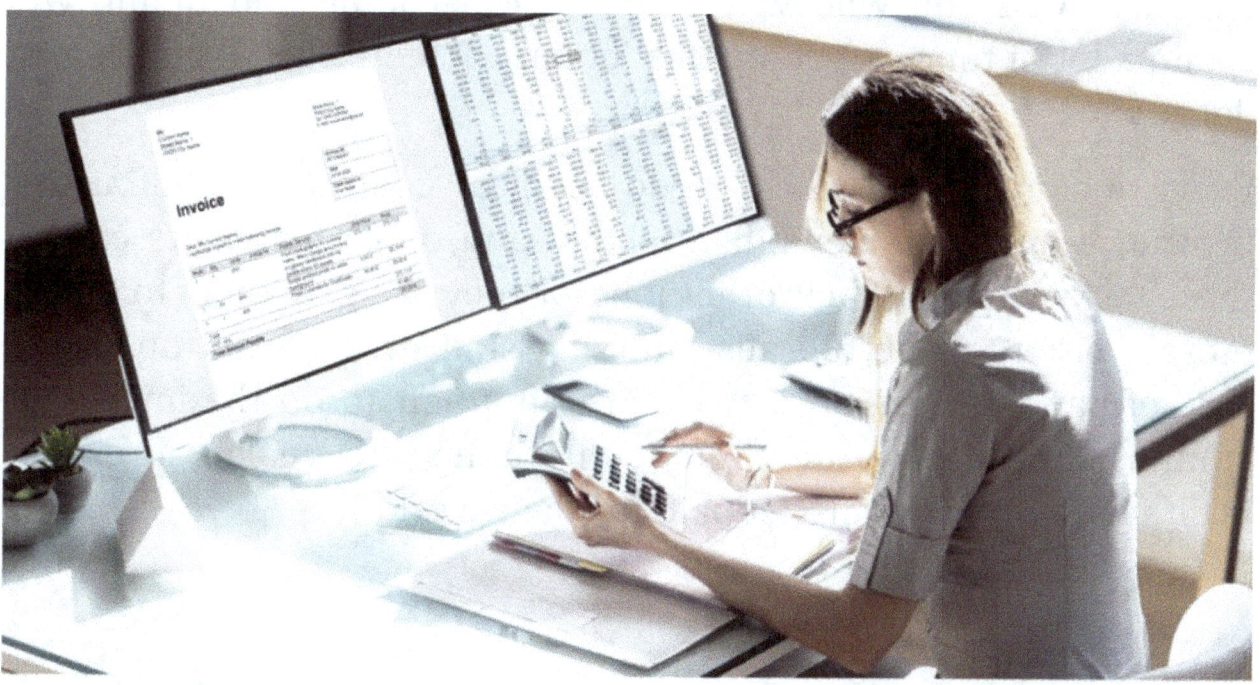

What exactly does this imply?

A coding and billing expert is in charge of the healthcare facility's insurance payments, billing, and transactions. Every day, a medical coding and billing expert has to do the following:

1. Accurately coding tasks, procedures, evaluations, and treatments

2. Making bills or payment claims and mailing them
3. Not accepting claims and correcting them
4. Paying attention to bills
5. Talking to patients and insurance companies about unpaid bills
6. Management of electronic health records
7. Following HIPPA rules for keeping records
8. Using medical billing tools to send bills and ask patients for payment
9. Management of medical billing systems

Even though these people often work in the same healthcare facility as patients, they usually do their jobs in an office rather than with patients. A person who works in medical coding and billing will spend a lot of time at a computer looking at, entering, and changing data.

Every medical facility has to do medical coding and billing for insurance and customer bills. Doctors and office managers can do these tasks on top of their other jobs, or they can give them to one or more workers to do. Because nursing staff are focused on taking care of patients, trained experts are often left to do the important administrative work of coding and billing to make sure that healthcare professionals get paid for their work.

CAN ONE PERSON TAKE UP BOTH JOBS

Medical billing and medical coding are two different jobs. There are different types of healthcare companies. Some hire one person to do both jobs, while others hire a biller and a writer separately. As I already said, each job comes with its own set of duties. Someone can be both a medical writer and a medical biller at the same time. It depends on the healthcare center chosen or the person whose job it is to see if they can do both.

CHAPTER FIVE: HOW TO BECOME A MEDICAL BILLER AND CODER

By taking online classes or going to college workshops, both medical coders and medical billers can get their certification in as little as seven months. Check to see what credentials the school offering the training has. Look for a course that teaches anatomy, medical terms, basic math, office management, computer software, and how to stay organized. All of these classes will help you get ready for your certification test and make sure you pass it.

Most people who work in this field get certified as either a Certified Professional Coder (CPC) or a Certified Coding Specialist (CCP). This makes them more marketable to employers. AAPC.com says that people with extra or advanced diplomas make up to $65,643. Getting more diplomas, a bachelor's degree or a master's degree may be helpful if you want to continue your schooling.

BECOMING A MEDICAL CODER

To get new job opportunities and promote yourself as a skilled expert, getting certified as a medical coder is a must. Medical writers don't have to be certified to do their jobs, but getting certified may help them advance and make more money. There are some important steps you should take if you want to become a qualified medical writer, no matter how much experience you have or how new you are to the field. Here are some ways to learn how to code medical records:

Obtain a diploma from a high school. The only educational requirement to become a medical coder is to finish high school. It might be helpful to take medical coding classes in high school along with math, science, typing, and other computer skills. Anatomy, chemistry, and medical terms should also be known to you.

Consider pursuing a college education. An associate's or bachelor's degree can help you move up in your career as a medical coder, but it's not required. It usually takes two years to get an associate's degree and four years to get a bachelor's degree. Getting a college degree will help you move up and be successful in your career. You might want to get a degree in health information systems or hospital management. Along with clinical coding classes, a graduate school will include classes in basic subjects.

Select a medical coding course. Several community colleges offer medical coding bachelor's degrees or licenses. People can go to class in person, online, or a mix of the two. The American Health Information Management Association (AHIMA) or the American Academy of Professional Coders (AAPC) should have accepted the school you choose. Each of these groups has a list of approved programs on their website.

Find out how many of their students pass the medical coding licensing exams and if they help students find jobs. An associate's degree program is better than a diploma program if you want to go to a four-year college to finish your education. Along those lines, you should also find out which classes you can take at another school.

Keep an eye out for for-profit universities and job training programs. For-profit universities also offer medical coding classes, and they usually have programs that work well for older students and students who already have full-time jobs. Often, these schools cost more than nearby colleges in the area. There are also fewer services to help students and help find jobs at these schools. A number of these schools also give out false information about their qualification.

Become a member of a professional group. Professional groups are a great way to learn about the field, connect with other medical coders, find job openings, and stay up to date on new developments. All over the United States, you can find local members of these groups. The American Academy of Professional Coders (AAPC) and the American Health Information Management Association (AHIMA) are two groups that medical coders can join.

WORK EXPERIENCE

The number of skills and experience a company wants will depend on how hard the job is and what it needs. It's usually better to have at least some work experience but don't let the fact that you don't have any experience stop you from applying if you've been taught how to do all the necessary jobs well. Most of the time, the following are the requirements:

1. A high school diploma is required.
2. An associate's degree in business or accountancy is normally required, with a degree in Business Management, Accounting, or Health Care Administration desirable.
3. A minimum of 1 to 3 years of medical office experience is required.

ADVANCED MEDICAL CODING CERTIFICATIONS

In the past few years, medical coding has become trickier. Medical coders who are trained in a specialty area may be best able to meet the needs of today's healthcare system.

To get their AAPC license, medical coders have to take and pass specialized courses, gain experience in a certain area, and pass necessary tests. Certification is the official recognition of a professional's work, skills, and reasoning. It's a sign of difference that needs to be kept up by studying and getting better all the time. As a coder, you can get the following certifications:

Certified Professional Coder (CPC)

The CPC certification from the American Academy of Professional Coders is the highest level of certification in medical coding. It shows that you have world-class information that medical organizations all over the country value highly and give out freely.

The Certified Professional Coder (CPC) test is the last thing you need to do to get certified as a CPC. This is the highest level of physician-based medical coding in the world. By taking the CPC test and getting the right to add the CPC abbreviation to your name, you become a healthcare worker known for having reliable knowledge of qualified medical coding.

Certified Outpatient Coder (COC)

As more doctors choose to work for hospital groups instead of their practices, the need for qualified outpatient coders is rising. This makes getting a COC certification an even better job choice.

Companies will know you know about outpatient hospital coding if you pass the COC test, which tests your actual understanding of MS-DRGs, APCs, and billing level indicators. Students who get their COC license describe outpatient services in some situations, such as

1. Hospital Emergency Departments
2. Outpatient Therapy Departments
3. Dialysis Services
4. Outpatient Cancer Centers
5. Outpatient Radiology Departments
6. Ambulatory Surgery Centers
7. Outpatient Hospital Clinics

Certified Inpatient Coder (CIC)

Certified Inpatient Coder (CIC) is the only medical coding certification for hospitals and medical centers that works only on inpatient coding. The CIC checks that people know how to get information from health records for ICD-10-CM and ICD-10-PCS coding. The course also covers the Inpatient Prospective Payment System (IPPS) and Medicare Severity Diagnosis Related Groups (MS-DRGs) professionally.

You can work as a medical coder and biller in a hospital inpatient setting once you pass the CIC test. This is because the rules for medical coding and billing are always changing. If students pass the CIC exam, they will be able to write reports about the care given to inpatients in places like medical centers (critical care amenities), skilled nursing facilities (SNFs), critical access hospitals (CAHs), teaching hospitals, inpatient rehab facilities (IRFs), and long-term care hospitals (LTCHs).

Certified Risk Adjustment Coder (CRC)

Without risk adjustment coding to make sure that a full picture of each patient's state is gathered and reported on medical claims, healthcare insurance would not have the money or knowledge to give high-risk patients the medicine they need. The job of Certified Risk Adjustment Coders (CRCs) is to accurately rate patients' risks. This makes sure that patients get the best care possible and that doctors and healthcare insurance get paid fairly.

Students who get the CRC certificate have shown that they understand how complicated diseases are when they have long-term conditions and problems, as well as ICD-10-CM and risk-adjustment suggestions. Because they are CRCs, they know how to make sure that the medical record accurately shows the patient's health and includes all medically confirmed illnesses.

Specialty Medical Coding Certification

Professional groups, healthcare systems, and surgical centers depend on qualified medical specialty coders to keep their billing processes running smoothly. The specialty certification test is the best way for these organizations to trust a coder's skills. Companies usually pay specialty coders 11% more than non-specialized coders because specialty coding diplomas show that the person is good at the skills they need.

CAREER ADVANCEMENT

Professionals often set goals that help them move up in their jobs. You can set goals to get better at being a boss and coding, both of which will help you do well at work. It's possible to do better as a medical biller or writer. Here are some ideas.

1. Obtain further certificates

Medical billers and coders always have a license or an associate's degree in medical IT or medical coding. Make goals that will help you get more awards, which will show that you have more skills and qualifications. Take a look at these certificates:

- Certified Professional Coder
- Certified Outpatient Coder
- Specialty Coding Certification
- Certified Risk Adjustment Coder

2. Increase the number of people you know.

Making more contacts as a medical writer and biller will help you learn about new job opportunities and get better at what you do. You could set a long-term goal to meet a certain amount of new people every month to improve your networking. For example, to grow your relationship, you could set a long-term plan to talk to five new health workers every month.

3. Look for a mentor

You could get better at what you do and learn more about medical billing and coding from a guide. Your goal should be to find a guide within a certain amount of time. After that, think about how you could find a guide. Someone like a boss, neighbor, or teacher could be your guide. Some medical schools have mentorship programs, and the office may be able to put you in touch with a skilled medical writer.

4. Obtain favorable feedback

If your boss or coworkers give you good comments, it means you do good work. You might want to make it a goal to get positive feedback, which could help you move up in your job or get professional honors like employee awards. Good acknowledgment at work could come in the form of compliments and praise.

5. Educate ambitious medical coders and billers

As soon as you know enough about medical billing and coding, you can start teaching other pros in the field. By giving them good tips on coding methods and practices, you can help them feel more comfortable. You may be ready for a leadership role if you teach people how to become experts in coding.

6. Be in charge of a coding team

Make it your goal to be in charge of your medical billing and coding department. For example, this could show the management that you can grow in your job and that you have the skills to teach and assist other hackers. You should tell your team boss or supervisor that you want to try out for a leadership role once you know what your goal is. If the person in charge of your team isn't there all day, they may let you take over their duties.

7. Improve your abilities

It might be helpful to set a goal to improve all of your skills. Medical billers and coders frequently need to be good communicators, data inputters, technical experts, professionals, and computer savvy. Think about the different skills you could improve, and then do tasks that will help you get better at those skills. To get better at computers, for example, you might do a job that needs you to use your computer more often so that you can learn more about how to use coding software.

8. Enroll in professional development classes.

You could set a goal to finish a certain amount of training classes to learn more and get better at what you do. You might be able to get better at your job and get more done by taking medical billing and coding classes. You could also take development classes that will help you improve your "soft skills," like lessons on how to communicate or lead others.

9. Boost your productivity

You could give yourself the goal of becoming more efficient when you are billing and coding. You could do a better job during your shifts if you were more efficient. Here is an example of how long it usually takes to do basic billing and coding. Then, set a goal to speed up by ten to twenty seconds. You can keep setting new goals for efficiency until you're happy with how fast you're billing and coding.

10. Take on the role of a mentor

You could help someone who wants to become a medical biller or writer by being their guide. Setting this as a work goal could help you figure out where you want your job to go. It might be helpful to help a new worker at your company and give them tips on how to get better and reach their goals. Also, you could put them in touch with people in your network who can help them with their job. Tell the people in charge at your company that you want to be a guide. This might help them put you in touch with new billers and writers.

11. Acquire knowledge of many systems

Medical facilities frequently use different coding features and methods when storing patient data and information. You could improve your skills and knowledge by learning a range of methods and techniques. This could help you provide better care to your patients. If you know a lot of different coding systems, you can focus on just one, or you can keep using all of them equally, based on what your company needs.

12. Become familiar with a variety of insurance schemes.

An important goal for medical billers and writers who work with patient insurance is to learn about all the different insurance systems out there. During the claims process, you may need to talk to insurance companies to keep track of surgeries and appointments with patients. You might want to look into how different insurance systems work and what they need, and you could also talk to your coworkers about these systems.

13. Make your workplace a happy place to work.

You might want to set goals to help make the workplace more pleasant. Medical buildings can be busy places, so it's important to have a nice place to work so that employees don't get too stressed out. Make friends with your coworkers and push them to ask you questions about how billing and coding work to make the workplace a better place to be. Also, try to help your coworkers solve any problems they may be having while filing claims or coding medical services.

14. Teach a course on medical billing and coding

With the right number of experiences in the billing and coding field, you can use what you learned on the job to teach a course. Your tips and strategies could help new billers and coders who don't have as much experience. You should think about the things you've learned from working in the field. Share your ways of talking to people, like if you learned how to quickly answer customers' common billing questions.

15. Push yourself to do things you're not used to.

You might want to get a job that will change your routine. You might learn new coding skills or methods that you didn't know about before. If you are happy working as a billing and coding clerk at a small medical facility, you might want to look for a job at a big medical center.

16. Practice being proactive.

Being proactive is important if you want to keep track of important information as a medical biller and coder. Goal-setting will help you become more aggressive, which will help you do better at work. Look for ways to be proactive in your daily tasks, like writing down a payment as soon as the facility receives it or getting in touch with a client as soon as you send them a bill.

17. Ascend to a position of leadership

Make it a goal to get to a top role. If you become a leader, you might be able to make more money and help your friends find decent jobs. Gaining a leadership role shows that you have the right skills and are ready to move up in your company. You could move up in your current company and become a manager, or you could leave for a better job at another company.

BECOMING A MEDICAL BILLER

The amount of time needed to become a medical biller depends on the job. Most college certificate programs last between 9 and 21 months or 2 to 4 quarters. The length of a bachelor's degree is four years, while the length of an associate's degree is two years.

Most people who want to become medical billers don't need a bachelor's degree, so it only takes them two years to become medical billers. When you go to school part-time, it usually takes longer to finish your degree.

Some fast-tracked classes only last a few months or even weeks. Medical billers can start looking for work as soon as they finish their training and get certified. The best time for each job seeker to do this is different. You can become a medical biller in the following ways:

Obtain a diploma from a high school (or equivalent).

If you have a high school diploma or a GED, you can look for entry-level jobs in medical billing. On the other hand, getting certified and going through a lot of training may give you more job options and help you make more money. To get into certificate/license programs and associate degrees, you need a high school diploma or the equivalent.

Enroll in a program for medical billing

The most common ways to get a job in medical billing are through training programs and associate degrees. New professionals can go to technical and trade schools.

You might be able to finish these classes in less than a year. They help people get ready for national coding certification tests and help people get their first jobs. There are online medical billing classes from some schools.

Companies like to hire people with an associate's degree, which can take up to two years to finish. A good foundation in general education can be found in an associate degree in medical terms, coding, and information technology.

Associate-level grads may be able to find work with insurance companies, the government, or health experts. It is common for students to move points from associate degree programs to bachelor degree programs.

Exams for certification must be passed.

Health care companies usually choose billers who have professional qualifications. These certificates show that the person knows a lot about difficult billing and follows the rules set by the government for coding. Getting certified could open up more job opportunities and raise your pay.

Look for work

It's common for schools that teach medical billing and coding to also help students find jobs. Students can get help from the career office with writing applications, practicing interview skills, and finding open jobs.

People applying for jobs should include information about any training and jobs they've had in the past. People can get information from AAPC about the states and cities with the best job opportunities and higher pay.

CHAPTER SIX: WHAT ARE THE QUALIFICATIONS FOR A SPECIALIST IN MEDICAL BILLING AND CODING?

The main skills needed to be a medical coding and billing expert are often the same, even though the job duties and requirements may be different. The most important thing is that you know the right codes, but other skills might help you get hired as well.

Medical Terminology

To code correctly, you need to know the basics of medical terms. This includes ideas like anatomy and chemistry, as well as terms for diagnosis and procedures. The process of billing and coding will go more smoothly if you know the medical terms that are used most often.

Math Fundamentals

You'll need to be able to do easy math to figure out the right billing numbers. Based on the numbers given, the billing system may fill out papers with the right amounts for insurance claims. However, you may still need to figure out how much patients owe or set up payment plans if needed.

Computer Proficiency

For medical billing and coding, you need to know a lot about computer networks and the most important medical tools. You'll also be better off if you can quickly learn new tools.

Communication Capabilities

As part of the medical billing process, patients may be called to ask for payment. For this part of the job, you need to be able to deal with others responsibly. Some people may be scared, irritated, or angry when they hear about medical problems and the high cost. Being able to communicate clearly can make these talks much easier.

Using Standard Office Equipment

In addition to knowing how to use computers, an expert needs to know how to use things like 10-key calculators, printers, copiers, scanners, phone lines, and so on. Since you've probably worked in an office before, you should know how to use these tools without any problems.

CERTIFICATION ORGANIZATION

There are a lot of groups that offer knowledge to help people understand and work in the medical billing and coding field. The following are a few of them. First, though, let's take a closer look at each group.

The AAPC (formerly the American Academy of Professional Coders) and the American Health Information Management Association are the two main certification organizations for medical coding and billing specialists (AHIMA). Medical coding at clinics is covered by AHIMA certification, whereas all other parties are covered by AAPC certification.

There are training resources, classes, and certificates from both the AAPC and the AHIMA. In addition, both groups offer the chance to network and get help from other members.

American Academy of Professional Coders

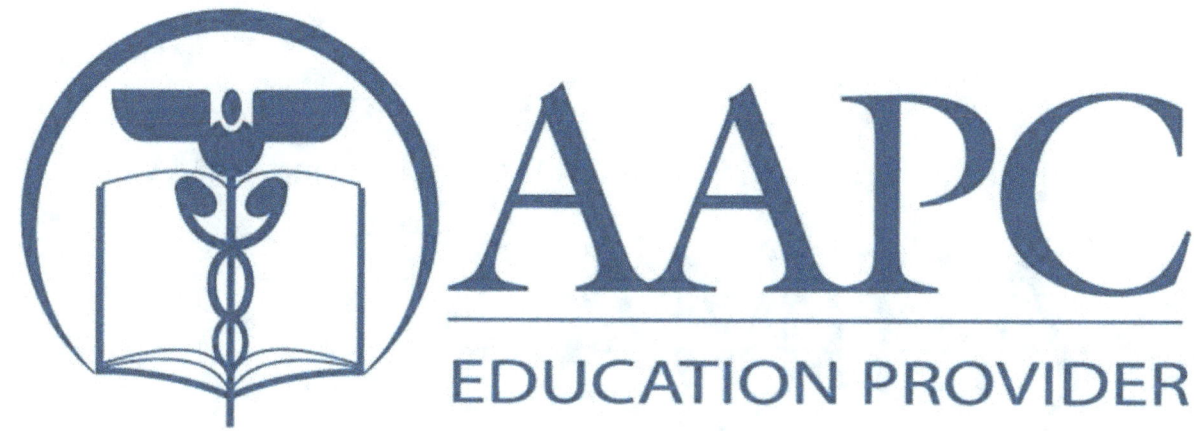

By giving students training, licensing, continuing education, networking opportunities, and job opportunities, AAPC raises the standards of medical coding by giving physician-based medical coders knowledge and career certification. It is the biggest group in the world that trains and certifies healthcare workers. Members work all over the world in areas like medical coding, billing, accounting, compliance, improving clinical paperwork, managing the revenue cycle, and running a practice.

Through job training, ongoing learning, and networking events, AAPC gives professionals in many fields many chances to improve their skills and advance in their careers. The American Medical Association (AAPC) was founded in 1988 with two main goals: to certify and train medical coders who work in doctors' offices and to improve the quality of coding by following accepted standards.

The AAPC is known for licensing both physician and hospital-based coders. Now, it's adding physical training and certification for healthcare lawyers and IT workers to its list of services. All over the United States, you can find AAPC training classes. The group also gives people the chance to keep learning and find work. The AAPC holds a national meeting every year so that its members can meet new people and learn new things. Regional conferences can do the same things as national conferences, and they usually work better too.

American Health Information Management Association (AHIMA)

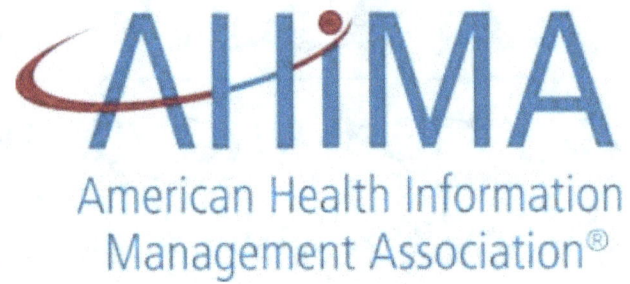

AHIMA is working with leading leaders in the field to set and support high, uniform standards for the use of electronic health records (EHRs). AHIMA is also ahead of the competition because it approves cutting-edge academic programs and career growth choices, such as full-time education.

Most of the people who get diplomas from AHIMA are medical coders who work in clinics. AHIMA was founded in 1928 with the main goal of making medical records better. Even though more and more people use electronic medical records, the organization still aims to be the most trustworthy source for medical records.

AHIMA is a well-known group for clinic and doctor writers. The group offers many training programs, holds a meeting every year, and holds workshops across the country that last several days. If you join AHIMA, you'll be able to get training and meet other people in your field throughout your job.

While AAPC gives out badges for apprentices, AHIMA only gives out skills for entry-level jobs. The AHIMA diplomas, on the other hand, are for people who are already very good at coding.

The Healthcare Billing and Management Association

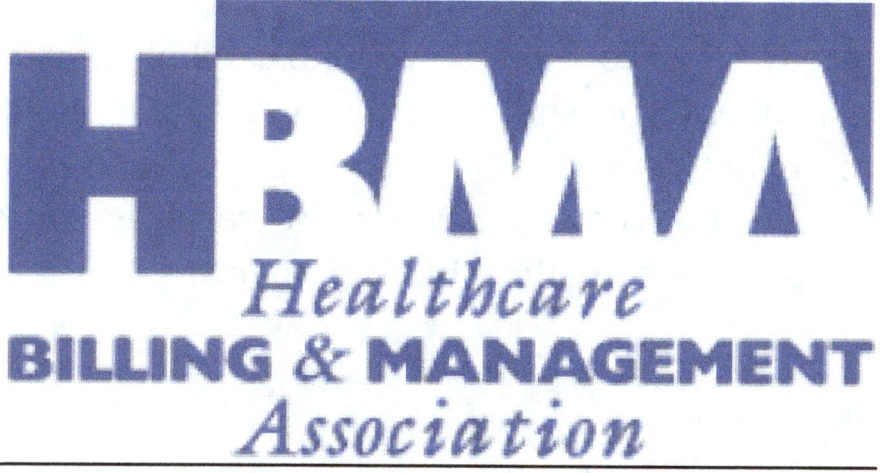

A small group of people came together in 1993 to start the HBMA. They saw the rich and successful as a way to work together to give the healthcare world a very professional picture.

In the US billing and coding business, the Healthcare Business Management Group (HBMA), a non-profit trade group for professionals, is a good choice. A lot of the first medical claims that go to the government and non-government payers in the country are made by members of the HBMA. Many times, the seller files these claims on their own, not through an HBMA partner company.

Some of the largest medical billing firms in the country are members of the HBMA, with over 1,000 employees who file millions of claims. However, the average HBMA member is a small to medium-sized business with 40 to 50 employees. Also, about half of the HBMA's members have clients in more than one state.

The private insurance industry and government groups that control or have an effect on the US healthcare system see HBMA as an expert in revenue cycle management (RCM). The HBMA pushes for the highest level of skill, ethics, and proper marketing methods in all areas of the healthcare field.

The HBMA is one of the most important services in the health field. You can ask us anything, from general questions about coding, study, and billing to the most detailed questions about medical billing. Members of the HBMA are professionals who can help you at any time with their vast knowledge. They might also be able to point you in the direction of people who have helped people with similar problems in the past. All of the HBMA's actions and services work together to keep you up to date on medical billing experts.

Medical Billers' Association (MAB)

In 1995, the Medical Association of Billers was the best group for teaching and accrediting people who work in medical billing and coding. The Council for Postsecondary Education has approved and accepted the MAB school. MAB is also a nationally registered business. So that more students can get certified, MAB works with other schools and training centers that are approved to offer the Certified Medical Billing Specialist certification test as part of their programs.

MAB's goal is to create medical billing and coding programs that are based on the values of dedication, motivation, skill, and honesty. To reach this goal, they try to find a mix between volunteering, learning, and improving the way they teach. In addition, they try to help medical communities across the country by giving advice and working together. They also help make and promote useful standards and build relationships with groups that are working toward the same goals.

The Professional Association of Healthcare Coding Specialists

This is a communication network and member support system that helps medical care coders work together better, make sure their work is correct, and get paid more. As PAHCS members learn more about coding ideas, changes to coding rules, and the experiences of other coders dealing with coding problems, they can easily code for maximum and honest pay.

PAHCS is a support group that helps its members talk to each other. Membership is open to all experts in medical coding, but the group's main purpose is to help medical coders. To work for this company, you have to fill out an application and pass a written test showing that you know how to use the mobile healthcare delivery system. If you're already certified by another group, you can apply for PAHCS certification by showing proof of your current certification and paying a registration and filing fee.

Medical Specialty Coding and Compliance Board (BMSC)

It's not well known that BMSC gives medical coders, compliance officers, and doctors training and certificates in medical coding. Persons who work in doctors' offices and people who give medical care at home can both get BMSC licenses. The academic standards for coding and compliance get harder with each level of certification. This means that BMSC certification helps hackers and other workers move up the ranks.

MEDICAL BILLING AND CODING CERTIFICATION

A business certification may help you get work because not all companies need certification to hire a medical coding and billing expert. You could make more money if you get certified in medical coding.

The Bureau of Labor Statistics says that the mean or average salary for a medical secretary in 2017 was $34,610 per year. This includes medical billers and writers. Still, you might be able to make more money if you get recognition in your field, like the AAPC's Certified Professional Coder (CPC®) title, and then work for a while. According to the 2017 AAPC Salary Survey, coders with thirteen years of experience or more and the CPC license made $54,106 a year.

Full CPC licensing needs job experience and other qualifications. However, people who pass the test but don't have experience may be given the title of CPC Apprentice (CPC-A). A CPC Apprentice can become a full CPC by showing proof of two years of experience or 80 contact hours of study to prepare them for coding and a year of experience. A mix of official schooling, licensing, and experience may help you make more money, especially as you move up to senior-level or management roles.

A medical office will usually ask for either experience or licensing when hiring a new billing and coding expert. Other offices may ask for (or prefer) candidates to have both. Getting a certificate or degree in medical billing and coding will help you learn what you need to know and get ready for the licensing test.

You must have at least one of the following medical billing and coding credentials to work as a medical coder:

- **Certified Professional Coder (CPC):** This title shows that you know how to use medical billing code sets and how to think about evaluation and management (E/M). You also need to show that you can follow rules and directions.

- **Certified Coding Specialist (CCS):** You must show a high level of commitment, coding skills, and professional ability in all medical situations. It's best for people who want to learn how to code for medical billing and coding.
- **Certified Coding Associate (CCA):** This credential shows that you know how to organize health data from patient information and have learned the method.

CERTIFICATION REQUIREMENTS

For entry-level jobs, you usually need to get certified in medical billing and coding or finish an associate's degree program. Students learn about ICD-9, CPT, DSM-IV, and HCPCS, among other methods for grouping things. Pathophysiology and medical terms are taught in the training.

They know about health insurance and the different types of public and private plans, such as Blue Cross/Blue Shield and Medicare. Also, medical writers need to know about the rules and morals of health insurance, medical billing, and the Health Insurance Portability and Accountability Act (HIPAA).

The US Bureau of Labor Statistics (BLS) says that companies usually want to hire people who have experience in the field. However, licensing is not necessary. Most people take the Certified Coding Assistant (CCA) test, which is taken by the American Health Information Management Association (AHIMA).

People usually take this test after they finish a training program. The Certified Coding Specialist (CCS) test can be taken by technicians who have worked as technicians for a few years. The test can be taken in a medical worker or care center setting.

HOW IMPORTANT ARE CERTIFICATIONS

There are jobs in medical billing and coding that don't require a professional license, but having one shows that you've been properly trained and have the knowledge and skills to be a good operator. This is why getting the certification is important:

Higher Income

The American Academy of Professional Coders (AAPC) says that certified professional coders (CPC) make 20% more than their non-certified coworkers.

Better job prospects

Even though the field of medical coding and billing is expected to grow at a faster-than-average rate of 15% by 2024, it is still a very competitive one. Most companies want to hire workers who have at least one qualification or can quickly get one after starting work.

Chances for advancement

Certification, especially in some coding areas, makes it easier for workers to move up in their careers and shows companies that they are dedicated to continuing to learn and the field as a whole. This kind of dedication pays off. In fact, in 2015, AAPC members with two or more qualifications made 24.5% more than those with only one. People who had three or more diplomas made about 40% more than people who only had one.

Business connections

Membership in organizations that give certifications isn't usually needed to get certified, but it can help you meet other people who are also experts in medical coding and billing. Many opportunities can come from working with people and groups that value and respect professional qualifications and schooling.

Personal Growth

Not only does passing a certification test open up job possibilities, but it also opens up options for personal growth. Professionals who are certified may be sure that they are doing their job right, and certification training can lead to new training and expert progress.

MEDICAL BILLING AND CODING SKILLS

You need to have a lot of different traits and skills to be a good medical billing and coding worker.

Organizational Skills

As a medical billing and coding worker, you may have to deal with a lot of information from different doctors or places. It's important to keep all of your papers separate and make sure you can easily get to the information. The most important thing you can do is make sure your work is right and that your bosses get their files on time.

A Basic Knowledge of Human Anatomy and Physiology

Physiology is the study of how the body works, while anatomy is the study of how the body is put together. If you understand these things, you'll be able to read and understand important medical papers that your boss gives you to handle. It's very important to understand what a doctor is saying.

Discretion

As someone who works in medical billing and coding, you will be in charge of doctors' patient information. You mustn't tell anyone else what you are doing because that would be breaching secrecy. If you talk about your job, you could get in trouble with the law.

Dependability

It is very important to look over papers correctly and on time. People who work with insurance companies, doctors, and patients must be able to trust the information in the records they keep. To get everything done on time, you need to decide how much work you can handle.

Good Typing Capabilities

To keep up with the fast-paced world of health care, you'll need to be able to type quickly and correctly. It's easy to learn how to type quickly if you've never done it before, and you can get faster with practice. You might want to sign up for free online typing classes if you want to improve your typing skills. You might be able to improve your speed by taking typing classes. This will help you do a better job and be more valued by your boss.

Strong Writing Capabilities

Being able to type quickly isn't enough. You also need to be able to work with words and put together correct grammar lines. You will make your boss dislike you if you make a lot of mistakes.

Cooperation skill

Medical billers and coders work well with others because they know how to talk to them and get along with them. These skills are used when working with other people, patients, and other healthcare workers. Teamwork produces beneficial outcomes like accurate treatment records and billing bills. Top medical billing and coding licenses help people work together better by giving them group projects.

Adaptability

Medical billers and writers need to be able to quickly adapt to new rules. These changes include problems that come up out of the blue, more work, or working extra hours. Despite having this much freedom, medical billers and writers are less likely to make careless mistakes when they are under stress. Their skills could be put to use in many areas.

Attention to Detail

People who focus on the details are less likely to make mistakes. This leads to better results for patients and correct billing records. Medical billing and coding workshops give students feedback that is specific to their needs. This helps workers become more focused at work. Some professionals may be able to improve how well they check their work twice.

Bookkeeping

A lot of the time, medical billers have to use their accounting skills. Part of accounting is dealing with financial information, like patient bills and payments. Employees often use bookkeeping to figure out their insurance bills and responsibilities. Bookkeepers with a lot of experience can spot mistakes that could hurt their patients or their business. An important part of learning how to do accounting is paying close attention to facts and numbers.

Accuracy

Medical billing or coding mistakes can cause delays in care or incorrect patient costs. Workers may keep their work accurate if they check it twice and don't rush through jobs that need to be done. As they do the coding and billing tasks, people working on their certificates and degrees learn more about accuracy and good business practices.

Technology Skills

People who work in medical billing and coding are often asked to use technology at work. The specific programs and apps that each company uses may be different, but the software usually lets users do the same basic things.

Below are some of the technical skills that are generally required to work in medical billing and coding, according to O*NET OnLine, a BLS database of occupational information:

1. Software for accounting
2. Software for billing
3. Software for data entering
4. User interface and query software for databases
5. Software for coding medical conditions
6. Software for coding medical procedures
7. Software for word processing
8. Software for the medical field
9. EHR (electronic health record) software
10. The Healthcare Common Procedure Coding System (HCPCS)

You can learn some of the basic tools and skills you need for a job in medical billing and coding while you are in school, but you may also learn them on the job.

CHAPTER SEVEN: HOW TO SELECT AND PREPARE FOR CERTIFICATION MEDICAL CODE

Before you start medical billing and coding school, take some time to think about your other options and pick the one that fits your needs the best. You could start by looking for medical billing and coding jobs in your area to find out what skills companies are looking for.

Once you know what the normal job requirements are, you should be able to figure out if you want to go to medical billing and coding school. These questions will help you choose which degree to get:

1. How does your everyday life look?
2. Do you think you'll have time to go to a nearby school, or would Internet classes work better for you?
3. Will you be ready for certification in your field after the program?
4. Is it possible to get individualized help through the program?
5. Will the school help you learn what you need to know and get the experience you need to start working as a medical billing and coding specialist?
6. What kind of hands-on training with medical coding tools does the school offer?
7. Will the training cover things that are often asked on certification exams in the field?
8. Can the school help me write my resume or get ready for an interview?
9. Does the school help people look for jobs?
10. What kinds of money-saving options are there for kids who need them?

Right after you answer these questions and pick a school, you'll need to start your first classes and get your certifications.

SELECTING THE RIGHT CERTIFICATION

You shouldn't feel alone in your plans to work in this field in the years to come. When you're finally ready to start your career, you'll be up against a lot of other people who have seen this possibility too. How can you make yourself stand out from other applicants and impress possible employers? The answer is to get a license before starting the job. Your career goals and what a potential company may want will mostly decide what kind of license you need in the end.

AHIMA says that certified coding specialists work in hospitals with patient records, while coders who want to become certified as a certified coding specialist-physician work in doctor's offices or specialized clinics. Keep in mind that some of these certificates have specific testing requirements, so the way you get them may not be the same as the way someone else does it.

Before certification, finish a medical billing and coding curriculum.

The licensing tests for all of the above-mentioned focus areas will test how well you can understand and do the duties and tasks that come with your job. A practice test can help you get ready for this kind of test. You will learn medical terms, circulation and venous systems, muscle systems, and industrial software.

Each license is different and has its own set of requirements for people who want to get it. As an example, AHIMA says that to become a qualified coding expert, a person must either have experience, a degree in coding, or learning that includes specific classes. The Certified Coding Specialist test has 97 multiple-choice questions and 8 medical cases. Once you're done with your training, you can look for the license that will help you reach your career goals.

Get certified before enrolling in medical billing classes.

Is it possible to get certified in medical billing and coding without first going through a training program? Yes, but you will have to do a lot of individual study first. The 150 multiple-choice questions on the AAPC licensure test cover a lot of material, such as CPT numbers, coding rules, medical jargon, anatomy, and more. Even after that, you'll still need two years of experience in medical coding to get qualified by the AAPC.

Getting through an advanced training program can help you feel better about yourself and get ready for the certification test. Some colleges even offer open course plans so that students can work and gain experience while getting a more advanced education.

Making a choice

There are several ways to get certified in medical billing and coding. It's very important to choose the best path for you based on your work experience and how you learn.

CHAPTER EIGHT: HOW LONG WILL IT TAKE TO BE A MEDICAL CODER?

How you get through the process is the main thing that determines how long it takes to become a medical writer. The length of the program will tell you how long it will take to get a certificate, diploma, or degree.

You can finish some certificate programs in less than a year. You should be able to finish an associate degree program and get your degree in less than two years if you want to do so.

You'll need to set aside extra time to take the test and meet the other requirements if you want to get CPC recognition. If you pass the test but don't have enough work experience to become a full CPC, you will be called a CPC Apprentice (CPC-A) until you show proof of your studies and/or work experience.

IS MEDICAL BILLING AND CODING THE RIGHT CAREER FOR YOU?

There are some things to think about when choosing a career path. Make sure to do your homework and ask all the right questions if you're thinking about a career in medical billing and coding.

You should find out how much the job pays, what it entails, and how the field is expected to grow in the coming years. But besides the job future and work setting, other things may affect how happy you are with your medical billing and coding job.

Take some time to think about these questions to find out if a job in medical billing and coding is right for you:

1. Can I follow the steps to the document?
2. Is it possible for me to keep patient information secret and keep their anonymity?
3. How safe is it for me to use tech?
4. Was it possible for me to work at a computer for a long time?
5. Do I get along with other people?
6. Is it possible for me to stay calm during tough times like billing problems?
7. I can keep my records in order.
8. Are my people skills good enough for me to talk to coworkers, patients, and insurance companies undoubtedly?
9. Do I pay attention to every little thing?

If you said "**yes**" to any of the questions above, you might be good at medical billing and coding.

CHAPTER NINE: REASONS TO BEGIN A CAREER IN MEDICAL BILLING AND CODING

1. Medical Billing and Coding is a Rewarding Career.

What number of people directly help each other every day? The sense of success you'll feel at the end of your shift is one of the best things about working in healthcare.

Medical billing and coding experts are important members of any healthcare team. Their job is very important for keeping costs down, preventing medical mistakes, and making sure that patients' health records are properly organized and recorded. Also, medical billing and coding offer the best mix of freedom and work-life balance.

2. The Medical Billing and Coding Industry is a Fast-Paced Industry

Over time, medical billing and coding have changed along with the healthcare business as a whole. This is mostly because of the use of electronic health records (EHRs) and other modern software tools for medical billing and coding.

This not only makes it easier to share and use medical records about patients, but it also cuts costs and gets rid of common mistakes. Medical billing and coding experts continue to be at the center of all significant changes because they can work in a fast-paced environment that requires constant learning and adaptation.

3. Billers and Coders in The Medical Field Has No Need to Attend Medical School

There is a great way to work in the medical field without going to school for years: medical billing and coding. Training for medical billers and writers can be over in just a few months.

Aside from that, medical billing and coding degrees are thought to be much less expensive than medical school. You won't have to pay back any loans or funds to get a head start on your job. This makes the job perfect for people in their forties or fifties who want to change careers but still need to support their families financially.

4. Medical Coding Errors/Mistakes Can Be Life-Saving

People who are good at paperwork are often left out of healthcare jobs that save lives. On the other hand, these people do a lot to keep people alive.

For example, if an incorrect code leads to the wrong care, it could be very bad if medical coding mistakes happen. Also, common billing mistakes can make it impossible to prove insurance benefits, which can cause a lot of damage and long wait times.

Making sure that data is correct and up to date is part of the work that goes on behind the scenes to keep hospitals and clinics running and doing well. Being a medical billing and coding worker will also save lives because of this.

5. Medical coders and billers may work in a Variety of Settings.

People who are thinking about changing jobs often worry about their ability to find work. You could be a medical writer or biller in a hospital, clinic, care home, administrative support center, or even a medical lab. Because so many different companies need these specialists, you can expect a strong job market with lots of choices.

6. Medical billers and coders work with some of the most amazing people.

People who work in medical billing and coding may face some problems, but their jobs may be beneficial in many ways. The changing work setting and wide range of workers help with this.

Some great medical comedies, like "Scrubs," show nurses and doctors from a different point of view. Even though medicine is a serious job, you'll probably work with a group of people who are fun to be around and have their own unique (sometimes dark) sense of humor.

7. Medical billing and coding can be started in a few months.

Some college students or people in their 40s or 50s who want to change careers might not be able to dedicate four years to getting a medical degree. It takes less than a year to finish most medical billing and coding classes.

If you pass tests offered by the National Healthcare Association (NHA) or the American Health Information Management Association (AHIMA), you'll be ready to work in some healthcare settings.

8. At Work, Medical Billers and Coders Dress Comfortably

There aren't many people who like to wear expensive suits, ties, shoes, and other dress clothes every day. Those clothes are uncomfortable and not right for the summer. Working in healthcare is a great choice if you want something simple.

Some people who work in medical billing and coding have to wear clothes when they work in a hospital or lab. Even though scrubs are made to be comfortable, you might look great in them if you put in a little extra work.

9. There Are a Lot of Medical Coding and Billing Jobs Available

If you spend time and money getting training and licensing in medical billing and coding, you'll be able to get a job right away. We're happy to tell you some good news.

The Bureau of Labor Statistics (BLS) says that between 2019 and 2029, the need for medical billing and coding workers will grow by 8%, which is a lot faster than the national rate. This means that people who work in medical billing and coding in the US will have a lot of new job possibilities. Also, healthcare administration jobs are some of the most sought-after related health jobs.

10. Medical billers and coders provide remote assistance to patients.

The part of any job that involves working with clients (or patients) isn't always the most fun. If you want to help people but don't want to work directly with them, medical billing and coding is a great job for you.

People who work in this field usually do their jobs in the background, handling patient data and making sure that the right medical codes and treatments are logged. Most of these jobs are good for introverts, and they'll be happy to know that many companies also hire people who work from home!

11. There are a lot of medical billing and coding jobs that you may do from home.

Do you believe that medical billing and coding is hard? No matter how bad the day is, putting on your favorite sweatpants makes everything better.

Many companies let their workers do a lot of their work from home because of this. One great thing about the job is that it's flexible. This is great for young professionals who don't want to commute and busy moms who want to spend more time with their kids.

12. Shifts in medical billing and coding are adaptable.

Do you like getting up early or staying up late? You should work whenever you have the chance, right? There's always a need for a variety of plans because many places that hire people to do medical coding and billing, like hospitals, are open 24 hours a day, seven days a week. Most of the time, you can switch to a second or changing shift if you don't want to work from 9 to 5.

13. You Can Work as a Medical Biller and Coder While Traveling

You may have always wished it would be warm all year. The good news is that Los Angeles, New York, Chicago, and Dallas are the places in the United States with the most jobs for medical billers and coders.

In the United States, you can find work in almost any town or city if your partner has taken a job across the country. This chance could only come up once, so make the most of it!

14. You Have the Right to Call Yourself a "Coder"

As an expert in medical billing and coding, you are not the same as a software developer, but you could legally call yourself a "coder." Software developers use coding languages to make software. It's not hard to make your job title sound cool, even though coding is all about finding and writing the right codes for medical problems.

15. In Medical Billing and Coding, there Is Room for Advancement

Being stuck in a job with no way to move up is not fun for anyone. You'll lose interest and be unhappy, and you'll start looking for another chance. If you get certified and work as a medical billing or coding expert, you'll be in the middle of the medical administration business. If you work as a hospital executive or in medical center management, you can learn more and maybe move up in your job.

16. Make a good living as a medical biller and coder.

In case you're still not sure if medical billing and coding is the right field for you, keep in mind that it's one of the 14 best-paying related health jobs in the US. Most people who worked in medical billing and coding in the US made more than $40,000 a year in 2019. For all jobs in the United States, this is more than the average. These numbers could be different depending on where you live, what kind of business you work for, and how long you've been working.

For example, the average income is best in the scientific and technological fields. Do you reside in the Garden State? If that sounds like you, you'll be happy to know that New Jersey pays the most for medical billing and coding, with an average yearly salary of $55,150!

CONCLUSION

Medical billing and coding is a vital component of the healthcare industry, bridging the gap between healthcare providers, patients, and insurance companies. Throughout this guide, we've covered the essential aspects of medical billing and coding, from understanding basic concepts to navigating advanced topics.

By mastering the processes of billing and coding, professionals can ensure that healthcare services are accurately recorded and billed, leading to efficient and effective healthcare delivery. The importance of compliance with regulations such as HIPAA and the Affordable Care Act cannot be overstated, as these laws help maintain the integrity and legality of billing and coding practices.

As the healthcare industry continues to evolve, the role of medical billers and coders will remain crucial. Whether you're just starting in this field or looking to advance your career, staying informed about the latest tools, technologies, and best practices is key to success.

We hope this guide has provided valuable insights and practical knowledge to help you navigate the world of medical billing and coding with confidence and expertise.

www.ingramcontent.com/pod-product-compliance
Lightning Source LLC
Chambersburg PA
CBHW082238220526
45479CB00005B/1272